HOMEMADE FACE MASK

DIY 15 different types of protective face mask for adults and children. guide complete with illustrations.

Table of Contents

Introduction

Chapter 1: What is a face mask

Chapter 2: Importance of face masks 1?
- *Disadvantages of face masks* 2?
- *Why Should You Make Your Own Mask?* 24

Chapter 3: Effectiveness of DIY face masks 26
- *CDC Recommendations for Wearing Homemade Face Masks* 28
- *What are the Best Materials for Homemade Masks?* 29
- *Rules to Wear a Mask* 35

Chapter 4: Washing your face masks 38
- *Wearer's protection* 40
- *How to Make Your Mask Bacteria Resistant* 41
- *How to donate your masks to help more people* 44

Chapter 5: Step by step guide to 15 DIY MASKS 47
- *Mask 1: D.I.Y N95 Respirator Mask* 47
- *Mask 2: Hand sewn face mask* 56
- *Mask 3: DIY Child Surgical Mask* 63
- *Mask 4: Mask Made of a Napkin* 65
- *Mask 5: Mask made with a gauze* 67
- *Mask 6: Double-layer face mask:* 69
- *Mask 7: Face mask with filter paper:* 72
- *Mask 9: Gas face mask* 78

Mask 10: Handkerchief or Bandana Face mask — 81
Mask 11: Face mask with cricut — 82
Mask 12: Easy No Sew Face Mask — 85
Mask 13: Using Paper Towels to Make Face Mask — 90
Mask 14: Homemade Cotton fabric face mask — 92
Mask 15: Home Made Mask with a Filter Pocket — 94

Conclusion — **100**

Introduction

Globally, everyone is keen to fight pandemics, and especially those that seem a threat to human health. The world has seen many people lose their lives because of the huge number of health-related problems as well as diseases that pose a threat to human life. The fact that these diseases are spreading so fast as world fire is undebatable. But do we wait till the last minute to face the edge of these critical and disastrous infections? We have seen a good number of people taking strict measures to curb and prevent the spread of these diseases and especially the viral ones. In some instances, it might sound strange to see people walking all over with face masks. Perhaps, in some areas, it is even unheard of. But what do we do when a critical disease hits? What do we do when a critical disease threatens to extinct human life? What do we do when the use of face masks is the only preventive measure to take? This is why most people will flood different stores to buy as many masks as they can. But buying of masks should not just be enough for that; ask yourself the kind and quality of mask you are buying. Usually, masks are worn by health professionals such as doctors, surgeons, and nurses when taking care of a patient. Of course, they do not just wear masks for no reason.

Basically, the masks are essential in two ways. First of all, they protect non-ill persons from getting sick by preventing them from exposure to different viruses. Two, masks are used from preventing further spread of viral diseases through sneezing and coughing.

With the rise of disease threats in the current world, governments and countries have taken a different turn in setting regulations to curb the spread of the diseases. Therefore, facemasks have become a piece of vital equipment in the war against viral diseases. The use of masks to prevent the spread of various diseases has raised various debatable topics from different professionals. It has now been an issue of concern while a group of doctors, scientists, and other professionals argue out the importance of face masks. On the other hand, others believe that there is no solid evidence to prove the essence of these face masks. Proponents of the essence of face masks believe that this equipment is essential in preventing the interpersonal spread of viral diseases. With most arguments against the use of face masks, a number of countries have adopted the use of face masks, and as a result, it has proved to be somehow effective. It might not be totally effective but at least proves some level of effectiveness. The use of face masks hasn't just started recently. Countries like China have been using face masks to prevent the spread of diseases, and the results have been seen to be productive. Other countries have followed suit. The nurses, surgeons, and other health professionals wear face masks because they have seen effectiveness in them. Definitely, there is the effectiveness with the use of face masks, and if there could be no effectiveness, then the health professionals, patients, and other personnel would find no reason for wearing them.

The rise of a terrible disease that requires the use of face masks instills tension, fear, and anxiety among many. It can instill even more fear when you find that face masks are missing from the stores. In which ways are masks believed to be efficient? How do they protect? Microbes in air and other surfaces often penetrate into the body's defensive system through the eyes, nose, and mouth. These microbes carry with them bacteria, viruses, and other harmful organisms. The use of face masks will, to some extent, prevent penetration of the microbes into the body. Therefore, it is through this that we can understand the use of face masks. But what step do you take if you cannot find a face mask or even afford one? The immediate step that should ring in your mind is designing your own mask, and this should come with various considerations of making the face mask.

Chapter 1: What is a face mask

Face mask is probably a word you've ever heard of. It's simply a piece of equipment that's used in preventing the spread of given diseases by covering the nose and mouth. Some other terms can also be used to define face masks. The terms are a dental mask, surgical mask, isolation mask or medical mask. These masks are unique and can cover the mouth and nose fully. Most if not all of them have rings or straps essential for holding them on ears.

Face masks come in many different brands.

In most cases, medical face masks are usually worn by medical personnel and perhaps expert researchers in the medical sector.

Apart from medical professionals, the remaining population can use face masks as well. This is done with the aim of preventing a massive spread of airborne diseases. Wearing of face masks is also essential in preventing intake of airborne particles from air pollution. Many people need to observe strict measures amid epidemics and diseases such as the novel coronavirus crisis which seems to be the world's major threat. Despite observance of several measures, the status of the person next to you is hidden as it takes a total of 14 days for symptoms to show up. Therefore, it's difficult to identify individuals carrying the virus. As a matter of fact, individuals should, therefore, shield themselves from this deadly virus through effective use of face masks.

Generally, face masks are essential protective requirements that can shield you from microbes, flu and the novel coronavirus disease, which is now posing a threat to the world. Carry your mask around, wear it as desired and help reduce the spread of coronavirus and other critical airborne diseases.

Face Veil

Technical markers of a decent face veil

Establishment

A number of particulate respirators are out in the market, and their appearance seems to fit well into the cautious methodology cover. Slight differences in their designs, nature and specifications sometimes tend to bring out undesirable functions. Mostly, respirators should undergo thorough tests and regulations before they are deemed fit for use. This chronicle, therefore, defines a number of specific qualifications that are geared towards ensuring the safety of a portion of the population which are administrative workers. Patients should also observe regulatory measures or rather be given these measures with the aim of assuring safety to the human administrative workers. When patients or infected persons observe these rules, there is a likelihood that no harmful viral or bacterial particles will be carried into the room through talks or wheezes.

Wear Time

The choice of respirators should strictly adhere to distinct guidelines. If you opt to have a respirator, ensure that it fits you well. Furthermore, the chosen respirator should be used carefully by using it in the desired time, environ and manner. In fact, respirators should ultimately be used in the most dangerous spots to ensure the greatest protection. Removing the respirator in the most critical spots means a reduction in its effectiveness. The cautious shroud is always worn to serve a specific procedure. The cloak is then disposed of accordingly after each method.

Testing

All respirators should adhere to speculations and criteria stated in the Code of Federal Regulations 42 CFR Part 84, especially in the US. To achieve the best in the test criteria, individual clients should clearly observe and review the guidelines. The U.S National Institute for Occupational Safety and Health(NIOSH) puts the channel capability test criteria into action. The criteria with "N95" channel media is as follows:

- The disintegration of sodium chloride test with center streamlined broadness atom with a mass of about 0.3

- 85 liter-per minute airflow pace

- Charge-slaughtered test disintegrated; and

- Preconditioning at 85% relative dampness (RH) and 38°C for 24 hours before testing. Normal tests for cautious/procedure shroud incorporate atom filtration adequacy (PFE), bacterial filtration capability (BFE), fluid check, differential weight, and instability. Each test is immediately delineated underneath.

Particulate Filtration Efficiency (PFE)

Social protection covers can be achieved through the quality PFE test. The test doesn't serve the purpose of respirator affirmation execution. The high PFE channel media of a cautious spread is of highly beneficial when the NIOSH N95 test procedure is incorporated. The results of the cautious shroud PFE testing and NIOSH filtration adequacy testing shouldn't be split further. The following are conditions that are critical for PFE testing:

- Disintegration of polystyrene latex circle test;

- A size of about 0.1;

- A 28-liter-per-minute airflow pace(ppm);

- Disintegration of the un-slaughtered test;

- Preconditioning should be avoided

Bacterial Filtration Efficiency (BFE)

The test focuses on giving an image of the limit of a cautious spread hence providing a suitable limit to huge particles evacuated by the wearer. The test doesn't serve as an equivalent of the managerial respirator filtration viability test. Furthermore, it doesn't explore the extent of security provided by the cautious spread. Usually, American Society of Testing and Materials (ASTM) methodology F2101-01 is the test used to assess BFE.

Fluid Resistance

Usually, this test is normally coordinated. It greatly relies on ASTM Test Method F 1862, "Assurance from Penetration by Manufactured Blood," which is typically based on the insurance of spread from blood squirted at it under fluctuating loads.

Differential Pressure (Delta-P)

The test is driven under some routines and is based on "Procedure 1 Military Specifications: Surgical Mask, nonessential (June 12, 1975)", MIL-M-36945C 4.4.1.1.1. It focuses on the weight of materials used hence a wait drop. The breathing ability is also another factor considered in this test.

Imperviousness to fire

There is always keen testing of cautious covers to ensure their suitability in any working room. The testing is majorly done to establish instability by class. According to the FDA, the most reasonable and effective instability materials for use should be of Class 1 and 2. The following rules have been passed by The U.S. Sustenance and Drug Administration (FDA) as a test of instability:

- UL 2154 End

Taking into account every precautionary measure, the cautious shroud is believed to set up a deterrent environment between the area of work and the wearer. They prevent or reduce the number of times the wearer with spitting and mucous problems from visiting a medical facility or undergoing a clinical apparatus test. Moreover, we can use to prevent fluids from appearing at the mouth or nose of the wearer. It is important to keep in mind that the cautious/technique cloak doesn't guarantee total respiratory protection despite the fact that it's a well attempted and a government-accepted respirator. It is also important for an FDA certified cautious/technique cover evaluated and affirmed by NIOSH as a particulate respirator. Such things are occasionally referred to as cautious N95, therapeutic or clinical respirator.

- The substance airborne centralization the wearer is linked to, and the substance world related introduction limit (OEL) are key in choosing respiratory protection for word related dangers.

- Biological administrators like diseases lack OELs. This is because it needs that supervisor to engage on heading available as well as picking the respirators. It is recommendable, and especially by the CDC that respirators with more confirmation be used in situations where exposure to microorganisms and contamination is a threat.

- The U.S. Word related Safety and Health Administration (OSHA) takes much responsibility in ensuring the word related to respirator use is adhered to. In fact, respirator use in any designated place must stick to the OSHA standard 29 CFR 1910.134.

- Respirators that fit tightly cannot go well with facial hair or any other thing that may interfere with the respirators seal to the face of the wearer.

Chapter 2: Importance of face masks

There is a great essence that comes with the use of face masks. Here are some of the ways in which masks are important:

- Masks are always useful during cold weather. When it's cold, a lot of people often suffer from different complications, for instance, influenza and cough. Germs are likely to spread easily from person to person. Therefore, masks are essential equipment for protecting the contraction of diseases from ill persons.

- Usually, most masks will fit your face well. During colder seasons, they are critical in trapping exhaled warm air and as a result maintaining a bearable facial temperature.

- In most cases, we've experienced bad odors, and masks can be a remedy for it.

- Towns have become terrible with an increase in the rate of pollution from automobiles, industries and factories. As a result, the air is contaminated with harmful particles. You will, therefore, need a way of handling these particles. Masks too are, to some extent, effective in preventing inhalation of such particles.

- Water droplets in the air may carry viral and bacterial agents. Masks are also essential in preventing these respiratory tract threats.

- Masks serve a key identification role. The masks, therefore, act as indicators of whether the wearer is ill or seeks to prevent infection. Those with masks colored on the outside are ill, and those with white masks on the outside are seeking to prevent the spread

- Masks are cost-friendly, affordable, easy to use and can be easily discarded after use.

- Health professionals use masks as essential health care equipment. The high number of patients they encounter on a daily basis forces them to adhere to proper sanitation guidelines.

- Masks serve as a better alternative for social distancing. Mostly, celebrities, as well as other personnel, wear masks to avoid contact with other people, especially when they have no feelings of doing so. They can also be good when you haven't worn any makeup.

Germs mostly facilitate the spread of dangerous diseases and viruses. These germs can be found in air, body or even contaminated surfaces. The germs can be transferred from the surface to surface through various means, and the most likely instance where the germs can be transferred is through sneezing and coughing. When a person who is infected coughs or sneezes, droplets containing these viruses are let into the air hence putting the people around in risk of being infected. But the droplets are too small to be seen by the naked eye. It is therefore essential to take great care considering that we know not of the components in the air around us. People mostly infect others through droplets which are a common medium through which diseases are spread. It is even fatal when the victim does not know about being sick as this can increase the rate of disease transmission from person to person. It is believed that sneezing with the mouth uncovered has the capacity of spreading the droplets in the air for about 6 feet. Suppose you are not aware of being sick from a dangerous virus, for instance, coronavirus, then you opt to board a bus or train. Sneezing or even coughing without taking cautious measures in such an environment is definitely a guarantee that almost everyone will be infected. Particles of the virus will automatically travel a distance of 6 feet in the air, posing a threat of contraction of the virus by the people on the bus or train. The only exception would be people who are wearing medical face masks that shield them from the penetration of dangerous and harmful viruses. Wearing of face masks can, therefore, reduce the spread of novel critical viral or bacterial diseases.

Touching is also another means through which droplets are spread. Touching things here and there is definitely a culture people have adopted and made usual. But when a critical disease strikes and the need for washing hands a minute after the other arises, people find everything harder. It should be realized that covering your mouth when coughing or sneezing doesn't assure you to go on touching things with the belief that you don't have a disease to carry on from surface to surface. When you sneeze into your and fail to wash them, you'll likely touch surfaces and contaminate them. The outcome is that many people will have access to such surfaces and increase the rate of transmission of germs and viruses. Such transmission occurs especially on door knobs where every person touches the doorknob without understanding the possible microscopic organisms hanging on the doorknob.

Currently, pharmacies have seen all sorts of people chipping in with the aim of securing at least a mask in the urban areas. Most people go for a large number of masks as they use them and dispose them off after they become dirty. Generally, masks play an important role during the flu season and most especially when a terrible airborne disease hits. The masks help filter the air breathed into the lungs and act as a barrier to the entry of deadly viral organisms.

Areas that are often characterized by large masses of people are at a higher risk of spreading an airborne disease or any other disease like world fire. It is therefore clear that wearing masks in such areas can be of much help. Medical personnel from urban area advise that disposable masks are hygienic while the use of cotton masks require frequent washing. Masks should be thoroughly cleaned after use to remove blocked particles and germs that can easily get into the human body through inhalation. This will then render the masks useless as their intended purpose will not be met. There are various masks, and their buyers should make proper choices. General masks can play the role of preventing dust intake. Medical masks are mostly used by professionals and seem to be more effective.

The spread of diseases and viruses is majorly accelerated through droplets. Therefore, we should keep in mind that personal approach in preventing the spread is key. Prevention of spread comes with strict observance of regulations such as the use of hand sanitizers, washing hands frequently, wearing masks when ill among others.

Disadvantages of face masks

While most people focus on the advantageous side of the use of face masks, it is also important to note that masks have their own cons as well. As a matter of fact, medical masks have various downsides which you didn't expect they would have.

In most cases, masks fail to fit the entire mouth and nose region properly. With the unfitting mask, there is the possibility of bacteria and virus making way through the two openings hence making use of masks a disadvantage. Furthermore, the medical face masks don't guarantee that all viruses or harmful droplets will be filtered out as a way of effectively protecting the wearer.

Medical personnel also advise that it's not a must for healthy members of the healthy community members to wear masks every time but rather focus on working in a well-ventilated room, taking a proper balanced diet and regular appropriate exercises.

Claustrophobia is a common complication that can arise from the use of face masks. A person who has claustrophobia can have a rough time when using the mask because it enhances the feeling of uneasiness.

With the use of masks, people can find it difficult to communicate. Hinder communication from person to person.

They make eating and drinking impossible. There are impossibilities brought about with the use of face masks. The wearer will obviously need to remove the mask before undertaking a basic activity like eating and drinking. Most likely, the removed mask should be replaced immediately.

Enhanced aspiration risk. The use of masks can result in choking and suffocation hence the need for handling the well.

Why Should You Make Your Own Mask?

Dependency on the stores for provision of masks isn't bad after all. But have you considered designing and making your own mask? There are a number of reasons as to why you should make your own face masks. Here is an overview of the reasons behind making masks of your own:

- Reliance on supply chain or stores isn't guaranteed

- There is more control over the strength, comfort and effectiveness of face masks.

- Making personal masks lowers the burden off the supply chain. As a result, the manufactured masks in stores can be enough for the rest of the population as well as health professionals.

- The ability to make personal face masks can guarantee an endless supply of masks that are washable and reusable.

- By making your own face mask, then the health and safety of the entire family at large is at your stake when dangerous pandemic hits.

- You will be more assured of a plan B in a case where plan A fails.

- Making your own face masks reduces the risk associated with rushing for face masks and queuing at the stores.

- It's upon you to decide how the face mask will look. The color and design of your mask greatly rely on you, and therefore the likelihood of going for a face mask you dislike is reduced. Even in the midst of a pandemic, you can bring more fun to life by preparing unique designs of masks.

Having had a clear picture of why you should make a face mask of your own, let's head straight to understanding the effectiveness of face masks.

Chapter 3: Effectiveness of DIY face masks

The effectiveness of DIY face masks may not guarantee the protection provided by N95 masks, but they will essentially shield you from a range of airborne diseases. When you don't have these masks, the risk of getting infected is higher compared to when you have at least one. The CDC even recommends the use of scarfs by those who can't afford to make or buy a mask. This is because the scarfs tend to offer some protection as opposed to when having none.

The DIY face masks protect well when diseases pose a high risk of spreading from person to person. This book will provide a detailed guideline on how to make face masks that are effective, essential and protective in terms of personal health.

DIY face masks have undergone thorough testing to determine their effectiveness. To understand the extent to which these masks work, air was pumped through a range of face coverings. From the test, it was discovered that medical masks had a 65% capability of filtering out microparticles. On the other hand, the N95 masks had an outstanding 95%

capability. The outcome of different fabrics proved different results which were dependent on the type of fabric. It was also discovered that using a fabric singly seemed to be unproductive, ineffective and useless as there was a 1% capability of filtering out microparticles. Other materials seemed to work even better than surgical masks by filtering about 79% of microparticles.

Currently, there is no equivalent alternative to social distancing even with the manufacture of highest quality masks. It is arguably true that masks work effectively but are not guaranteed to be a perfect substitute for social distancing. Therefore, there shouldn't be high expectations with reliance on face masks as there are other better alternatives such as limiting movements as well as washing hands frequently. Restricting movement and washing hands frequently are, in fact, the major ways through which viruses such as coronavirus can be prevented. Let not homemade masks give you a false perception of total security against the virus. The masks help but can, at times, prove to be harmful. However, when making homemade masks, there are a good number of tips to put into consideration. These tips can enhance the performance of face masks in preventing the spread of a critical viral infection.

Always go for masks tied around ears rather than those with elastic bands. This is because those tied around ears can be easily adjusted to the face as opposed to those with elastic bands. Always avoid wearing wet masks as they are likely to enhance the rate through which viruses penetrate through. Ensure that masks are always clean before usage. More importantly, desist from using chemicals and other bleaching agents on your masks as they can bring about dire effects.

CDC Recommendations for Wearing Homemade Face Masks

CDC recommends that cloth face masks be worn in public along with observance of given distancing measures. But there are some areas or localities in which social distancing is a hard-to-maintain measure. Consider supermarkets and banks. They are often situated in an urban locality and serve as the greatest spots of disease transfer. It is, therefore, advisable to adopt the use of cloth coverings as a way of preventing a contagious disease from reaching its peaks.

The use of cloth coverings is also essential in lowering the spread of a given disease from an ill person to a healthy person. Therefore, low-cost fabrics can do better.

Children who are underage and especially below two years should not use improvised face masks. Persons with breathing difficulties and other related health issues should avoid using them as well.

What are the Best Materials for Homemade Masks?

Do we just take any other material and improvise or make our own face mask? The answer is definitely no. There are a number of excellent materials which can do better when making a homemade face mask. Consider pillowcases and cotton clothing or T-shirts. These can serve as good materials for homemade masks, but then, multiple layers are usually believed to offer the greatest protection. Addition of filters on face masks can also be a good idea. Just like any other parts of the mask, filters serve a common purpose of shielding the wearer from harmful particles and microscopic organisms without necessarily affecting breathing.

The use of masks depends on the number of times you change it. Change of masks plays a great role in determining the mask's efficiency. The filter for the masks should be positioned between two fabric layers purposely for preventing inhalation of filter materials.

Abrasive materials are dangerous to your skin. Always limit your exposure to these materials. Additionally, materials used in designing and making homemade face masks should not extrude fibers that can be inhaled. This ensures breathing without difficulties and prevents moisture and harmful particles from sticking on the mask. It is, therefore, critical to put several factors into consideration before rushing for materials required in making masks. Acceptable, quality and certified filters should be the best alternatives to go for. The acceptable masks are highly effective in preventing the penetration of dangerous microscopic droplets and also in enabling effective breathing. These masks contain materials that won't extrude their particles, therefore, lowering chances of inhalation of toxic microscopic materials.

It's also important to limit the exposure of your skin to abrasive materials that can cause irritation. In addition, it's important that the materials you use for your mask don't extrude fibers, to avoid inhaling them. This will secure unobstructed breathing without easy saturation with the particles and moisture. While choosing better materials to use for your masks, go for high-quality, certified filters. Certified filters don't allow microscopic droplets to pass and allow undisturbed breathing. In addition, they are made of materials that won't extrude their particles and reduce the chances of inhaling the synthetic material.

The same guidelines also suit with the use of coffee filters and vacuum cleaner bags. Air conditioner filters are also good and advisable for use but it's also better cease from using those made of fiberglass.

Other better alternatives for filter layers are non-woven synthetic materials such as wine bags. The difference between these materials and the N95 face masks results from their thickness and weave. Otherwise, both are made of similar materials. Non-woven polypropylene is firm and tough and can be considered effective for multiple use.

The less efficient materials include those that allow more particles to penetrate through them. For instance, coffee filters, paper towels and other materials allow these particles to pass through them easily. Furthermore, the materials cannot be washed and disinfected frequently. They are the choice you can go for when all other choices are exhausted. Coffee filters permit one-time use and are a better choice for enhancing functionality of face masks. Despite their ability, they are considered less essential. But they are also meaningful when it comes to preventing the spread of harmful microorganisms, viruses and bacteria. Generally, it's better to have at least a form of protection, regardless of what it is, provided that it's essential. Having no protection at all enhances the risk of transfer and spread of pathogenic diseases.

Mask Filters

Masks that have filters can be made differently basing on given strategies. A double-layered cloth mask with an added filter can significantly increase the likelihood of preventing pathogens from penetrating (Livingston et al., 2020). A HEPA set of filters is quite a better option to try before making a filter for your mask. The filter should be of size F1 and should enable creation of 15 feet of fabric with a breadth of 6 inches. A single filter should have pieces sized 16x8 inches.

A pack of filters should produce a total of 22 face masks. Carefully remove the filters from the bags and ensure no damage is caused. Always ensure the HEPA fabric is preserved by adhering to the following strategical procedure:

Cut out the ends of the filter, and cut out the pleats carefully

In the case where you find dried glue holding together fabric pieces, remove them with caution. Finally, remove a piece of HEPA fabric and get set to make a face mask.

It should be noted that materials used in making face masks are porous and delicate. Therefore, frequent handling can bring about damage. Though homemade filters may be considered less efficient, they play a greater protection role when used in face masks. Wearing a face mask without filters always enhances the risk of penetration of pathogens.

Are Cotton and Flannel the Best Materials?

With the use of pillowcases, research depicts that 600-thread count flannel and cotton fabrics can secure 60% filtration (Livingston et al., 2020). The fabrics can highly prevent harmful pathogens. Additionally, they are even more efficient with the use of multiple layers. At one point, you might opt to try household air filters. They are important as well but also come with downfalls. Some of the household air filters might have fiberglass, which can cause severe complications to lungs if inhaled.

In comparison to N95 masks and surgical masks, these masks tend to be less protective. However, they reduce the spread by protecting your immediate neighbor from contracting a disease you are carrying unknowingly. According to research, quilter's cotton also protects by supporting about 80% filtration. Also, avoid thicker materials as they can bring about difficulties in breathing.

According to filtration professionals, a minimum of two non-woven fabric layers is considerable. That's not enough. You will also need to uphold high maintenance and cleaning standards to ensure that your mask serves you better. Don't forget to thoroughly clean your hands before using the mask. After using the mask, you have to either throw it away or wash it well. Also, it is recommendable to wash the face and hands after using the mask.

During the design phase of your face mask, it is critical to put some factors into consideration. The space in between the nose and the chin should be minimized as possible. At the same time, ensure that the comfortability of the mask is intact.

Handing the masks also requires some skill. Always avoid touching the masks every time and restrict yourself from touching it during removal and wearing of the mask. Effective protection can also be acquired from a combination of 3D printed masks and furnace filters. Though effective to some degree, the combination doesn't assure that you cannot acquire or get the disease from an infected person.

Having known the underlying essence of homemade protective face masks, it is important to explore a number of designs that can be used in making face masks. Additionally, having knowledge of recommended materials, a number of unique designs can be made.

Rules to Wear a Mask

It is not just all about making your own mask, wearing it in any manner and assuring yourself safety. There are also guidelines that will guide you through effective ways of wearing your mask to ensure safety and protection.

Mask, just like any other health equipment, has a role to play. It's not just a piece of clothing or rather an ornament. It is a tool critical for protecting any individual from dangerous pathogens, viruses, bacteria and microorganisms floating in air and surfaces. Occasionally, people fail to adhere to guidelines revolving around the usage of masks. With masks, you will have to adhere to strict usage measures so as to see productive outcomes. Adhere to washing hands before and after wearing a mask. In fact, make it a habit.

Usually, masks should be worn in a period of about 2 to 6 hours. But there are cases where epidemics hit and everything seems to be dangerous. Furthermore, you can find yourself in an area such as hospital where the rate of spread of a critical airborne disease is high. In such cases, consider wearing your mask for less than two hours because the environment you are in has many infectious agents and therefore speedy contamination and infection. Your external environment is, therefore, a critical determinant of the duration for wearing your mask.

Always go for new masks once your usual masks are damaged or dirty. Ensure your hands are clean before and after wearing a new mask. Carefully dispose your damaged or dirty mask in the desired place such as a plastic wrap. After disposing it, wash your hands once more.

- Wearing of masks shouldn't be done while eating or drinking. It is important to ensure that no drinking and eating takes place when you are wearing a mask because doing so will render the mask useless as microbes and pathogens will easily find way into your body. It is also not advisable to set the mask aside while eating and drinking.

- Always ensure to wear your mask in crowded places and public areas. By doing so, you'll be reducing disease transmission rate from an unknown person.

- Avoid touching your masks when wearing it.

- Don't wear wet masks or change the mask once it becomes wet. Wet masks provide a perfect environment for pathogens hence putting the wearer of the mask at risk of getting infected.

- It is advisable to have highly fitting masks. An unfitting mask permits entry of pathogens through open spaces hence putting the wearer at risk.

- Remove your face mask carefully without grasping it wholly with your hand. Always use the ear loops for removal of masks.

- Do not reuse a mask you have always used.

- Avoid removing and returning bandages on a mask. By doing so, you will enhance the process of contamination.

- Use soap wash your hands regularly after removing a mask

- Ensure your mask is tight to fit your face but not tight to the extent of harming your skin

- You can use bandages with a mask for the sake of elongating the mask's duration. Always remove bandages after a period of 4 hours and wash them, dry them and iron them.

Chapter 4: Washing your face masks

Frequent washing of facemasks can really enhance the protection provided against harmful microorganisms. It is believed that washing of hands before and after removing your masks can highly prevent contamination from bacteria, viruses, and other pathogens. Handling your mask in the right manner also has some effectiveness in preventing contamination. It is usually advisable to use the elastic handle rather than handling the mask wholly. Always minimize the contacts on the surface of the mask and avoid squirming while wearing your mask. More importantly, it is advised that you dispose your mask in the right manner immediately after use. In a case where you don't want to discard the mask, always ensure to thoroughly clean it with efficient sterilizers to kill the present pathogens. If you find it hard to access an efficient sterilizer, you can wash your mask with soap and clean water because soap proves to wash away coronaviruses.

How to Use And Care For Your Mask

Care needs to be taken for every mask you wear. The following tips should be considered before using masks.

- Ensure proper washing of the mask before usage.
- Thoroughly wash your hands before putting the mask on
- Avoid reusing a mask without washing it
- Immediately remove wet or damp masks and substitute them with dry ones. Wash the wet ones and dry them for the next use.

When you want to remove a mask:

- Always use the mask's string or band when removing it. Avoid contact with the surface of the face mask.
- When using a string mask, untie the string above after untying the one below.
- Use at least forty seconds to thoroughly wash your hands in clean running water. Hand sanitizers with 60% alcohol content can also be a perfect alternative.
- Wash your face masks in soap solution after removing it.

Other Tips

- Always use your face mask while away from home. Avoid using it in the car or at home. Use the mask is crowded and public places where social distancing is hard to practice.

- Avoid removing your mask in public or in places where you cannot get water easily. Wait until you get home and remove your mask.

- For non-sewn face masks, always remove the inserts of paper towel before soaking your mask.

- Stay at home and avoid going to public places once you have symptoms such as cough, fever, or stuffy nose.

- Finally, only go out once you have a serious business or thing you want to do. Avoid unnecessary movements away from your home.

Wearer's protection

It is more important to strategize on operational procedures and clinical strategies that are geared towards countering the transmission of dangerous pathogens to the immediate staff. With the aim of determining the effectiveness of any given mask against harmful aerosolized agents, Weber et al. examined a number of masks for particle penetration via leakage or mouth. The research showed that surgical masks have a lower tendency of protecting different personnel from dangerous tiny particles.

Protection of the health staff from contamination is an issue that calls for attention. The health personnel often meet different patients and, therefore, are considered to be in the midst of high infection rates. According to a study conducted on 40 Hong Kong hospital workers with SARS, all workers used masks with a minimum of 95% filtration capacity. 28% used eye masks, while respirators were not used. It is through the study that we realize the inadequate defense provided by surgical masks against SARS. The research is considered the most efficient and well done as it's the only research that focuses on the health of health workers.

Various medical associations in the U.S and U.K believe that surgical masks don't provide quality protection to patients and well as the medical staff. Despite being partially effective, it's good for personnel in critical fields to adopt their use for the sake of lowering infection to some level.

How to Make Your Mask Bacteria Resistant

Masks can essentially be improved to counter bacteria through the addition of layers of essential oil. The reason for the use of essential oils is that they have properties that help counter microbial, septic and inflammatory effects. The oils generally perform basic body functions such as boosting the immune system as well as shielding you from adverse weather conditions and allergens. There are specific oils that are preferable in providing the best anti-inflammatory, antiseptic and antimicrobial properties. All you need is to apply a thin layer of these oils. The following are some of the oils:

Eucalyptus Oil:

This oil helps in treating cold and cough, and this explains why it's commonly used during winter season. Eucalyptus oil provides high resistance to bacteria, and addition of a layer to your mask can be a good idea.

Mint Oil:

The oil boasts a number of antibacterial properties. Additionally, it's a flavor that is loved by most people. An additional layer of mint oil to your mask enhances the mask's efficiency.

Tea tree oil:

It's an oil that has been in use for years and years. Usually, it's essential in treating respiratory diseases. Tea tree oil counters bacteria to a greater extent and can be an additional form of protection on your mask.

Juniper Oil:

This oil is rich in anti-inflammatory and anti-bacterial properties. Mostly, it essential when it comes to shortness of breath and cough. Applying a layer of this oil on your mask shields the mask from entry of pathogenic particles, which can be a danger to your body.

Carnation Oil:

Carnation oil is also a greater oil when it comes to fighting viruses. Just like other essential oils, it boasts antibacterial properties hence effective in fighting bacteria. Addition of this oil to your mask can enhance its effectiveness because it levels up the efficiency of the mask against bacteria and viruses.

Myrtle Oil:

Are you having issues such as cough and running nose? Worry not. Myrtle oil provides an immediate solution. The oil is powerful in fighting microbes, and application to your mask can bring about greater protection. The oil ensures no bacteria or virus penetrates the mask.

Essential Oils From Citrus Fruits:

Oils from citrus fruits also prove to be efficient. Oils obtained from fruits such as lemons and oranges are good in fighting bacteria and viruses. A combination with other oils is even much better, as it can bring more efficiency. Try on your mask and enjoy the results.

How to donate your masks to help more people

With the coronavirus crisis, the world has seen different places immediately turn into areas for donation of masks. The immediate change has occurred as a way of handling the virus with total preparedness. Thanks to the personnel on the frontline of distributing free masks as a way of reducing the spread of this viral disease.

Additionally, huge business enterprises, companies, and organizations have come together to fight the virus, which is now the world's immediate enemy. The key thing here is to donate masks to save lives but not to donate them for popularity or to showcase the power of giving.

Donations should not necessarily be done in large amounts. We are not necessarily discouraging heavy donations because they help many persons. But consider a case where you can't afford large donations, yet you need to give out to a larger extent. In short, you don't have to strain yourself, but all you need is to focus on donating the little you have. In this section, you will now understand where to direct your mask donations.

Due to their effectiveness, N95 masks are in demand. Mostly, they are used by the medical staff, but access to them is slowly improving, and some will gradually have access to them. It is important to consider that not everyone can have access to these masks, and therefore, a better option is the fabric ones. Everyone has to cover their face, and therefore, critical considerations should be put in place to pick out the best masks for donation.

Donating is one important task. But the choice of masks for donation is even much better.

The criteria of choosing masks for donation is as follows:

- The masks should have a wire at the top, and the wire should go over your nose without hindering breathing.

- The masks should have an observable front and back. There should be a distinction between the front and back, and these can be done through styling or coloring.

- Materials used should be of cotton and should permit reusability and ability to wash.

- Though paper masks are generally unsuitable, they can be a good substitute during road jam.

- Ensure to have a tightly woven fabric mask for the sake of assured efficiency.

Having known the kind of masks to go, let's understand where you can donate them.

The United States has many localities. It is, therefore, better to contact hospitals to understand their need for face masks. Contacts can be done via email or phone.

Chapter 5: Step by step guide to 15 DIY MASKS

Mask 1: D.I.Y N95 Respirator Mask

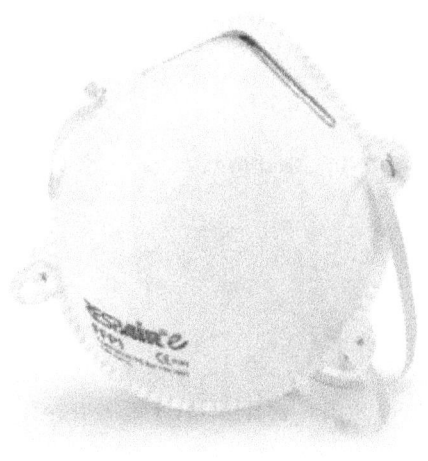

Designing a DIY N95 respirator mask requires that you are an expert in sewing and also skillful in some way. The complexity that comes with the design of this kind of mask doesn't require haphazard preparation. To come up with an efficient mask of this kind, you will have to set aside enough time and put in more effort to achieve the 95% efficiency level.

Equipment required:

- A sizeable woman's bra (the size varies with different faces)
- Citric acid
- Ruler and marker
- 1 Metal office fastener
- Craft glue
- Some soft material (any type and color)
- Unused coffee filters
- Needle, thread and sewing machine
- Material scissors

Directions:

1. Thoroughly clean and disinfect the surface and equipment to be used. Specifically, clean the scissors and needle to prevent the transfer of dirt onto the mask when making it.
2. Take the bra and cut around its cups and separate them from the straps. Ensure to gently cut the straps and reserve them for use at a later stage. Dispose everything accordingly and retain the arm straps and the bra cups.
3. In a case where you meet an underwire in the bra, you will have to remove it. To do so, make a tiny hole at one end close to the position of the underwire. Try to push the tip of the underwire out and remove the

whole thing. Having removed the underwire, you have to get ready to make your mask. Ensure that the bra holds a resemblance of a face mask once it's set aside on its own. Also, ensure it is rounded by your chin and should have a point for your nose. Therefore, to make a mask out of it, fold the bra halfway and ensure all corners are touching each other. Using a ruler, locate three inches upwards from the base of the bra. Measure an inch along the bottom right from the bottom corner. Using a ruler and a marker, draw a line to join the marks.

4. Sew the two sides of the bra along the line drawn. To achieve this, use your needle or sewing machine along with a thread. You can consider sewing it severally to ensure firmness and stiffness. After sewing, make a knot and ensure the stitches are well done. Turn the bra inside out to ensure the stitched side is on the inside. However, the seam should be visible. You can now try fitting the mask on your face. If the mask seems bigger, adjust it accordingly by sewing another line that is a bit closer to your face. However, ensure that its well-fitting for an average adult. If you are satisfied with your mask, cut off the sewn already sewn edges, ensuring to leave some space between the sewn line and where you cut from.

5. Glue the metal office fastener on the outside of the bra. Ensure the pointed tip is by your nose and the metal office fastener centered there. To give your mask some more desirable shape, you can slightly bend it to make the mask fit the shape of your nose. Add a dollop of craft glue on the metal piece center and put it on the tip of the bra below the sharp point. Test the mask on your face again and press down the metal piece until it attains the shape of your nose. Glue the edges and outside of the bra and leave the mask to dry.

6. You can prepare your coffee filter as the glue dries. To do so, cut the coffee filter to fit into the inside of the bra without ease. Put the citric acid inside your coffee filter. Citric acid is essential for creating a favorable environment with a suitable pH against bacteria and viruses. Usually, the acid is used in N95 respirator masks. Reserve your coffee filters for later use.

7. After preparing the coffee filters, you will be required to stitch the material on the inside and outside of the bra. Ensure the material is thin and light. The addition of thicker materials means there can be problems resulting in breathing through the mask. Let the material be of your preferred color as it ensures uniqueness in your mask. Shape the material into the

exact design of the bra and stitch it to the edges of the bra using a needle or sewing machine. Ensure to sew the material until it fits tightly around the mask. Cut off loose edges when done.

8. Prepare another material to be used on the inside of the mask. Let it be quite bigger than the mask so that it's loosely fitting to allow face comfortability. The material should also be thin and allow breathability. You can now sew the material around the inside edges of the mask. You can use a needle or sewing machine; the choice is yours. Ensure the stitch is strong. Carefully sew the sides and around the bottom, leaving the top open. Cut off the top material until to ensure it isn't a bother to you. You will now remain with a pocket inside your mask.

9. Take the initially reserved coffee filter and put it inside the pocket. The coffee filter will serve similar functionality to the in N95 respirator and will enable the killing of about 95% of microbes. Remember to dispose the coffee filter well after each use. Immediately replace it with a new one after discarding it.

10. You now have to make a strap for your mask. Trim the edges of one of the arm straps to acquire the desired cut. Resize it to fit your head. Adjust the strap

to its smallest setting and test it around your head. Ensure its fit to reach the front of your ear. In case it's too big, cut it to a desired extent. Always readjust it if it seems too small. Using a needle or a sewing machine, sew the end of the strap onto each side of the mask. Always sew the ends to exact corners of your mask on each side of the face. Ensure the stitch is tough, clean, and strong. Always keep in mind that the adjustment of the strap faces outwards away from the head. As a result, there is an easier adjustment of the strap when using the mask.

11. After sewing the strap, you can now check the suitability and efficiency of your mask. Ensure that it properly fits around the bottom of your chin and ensures some comfortability when worn. Also, ensure no gaps appear around the cheeks, nose, or chin. Adjust the metal piece around your nose to fit the shape of your nose. Once you feel satisfied with everything on your mask, you can consider yourself having properly made a D.I.Y N95 respirator mask. Get ready for its use and even donate if possible.

The complexity that comes with this design of face mask requires that the maker is keen and observant during the process of making it. The mask involves a number of steps and materials that are unique and key in protecting the wearer from pathogens. The use of coffee filter and citric acid adds some value in protection and protects well just as an N95 face mask would protect.

The D.I.Y N95 respirator face masks can specifically be made for children and adults. The mask can work even much better with the use of smaller cup-size women bras. But if you need a bigger mask, you can use a large cup-size women bra. This design assures almost total protection to the wearer and, therefore, a good option for your family.

Considering that you have two cups from the bra, you can make two masks out of a single bra. What you require is to use one strap and one cup for each mask. It, therefore, proves to be an efficient way of making masks that will shield and protect you from harmful pathogens.

Mask 2: Hand sewn face mask

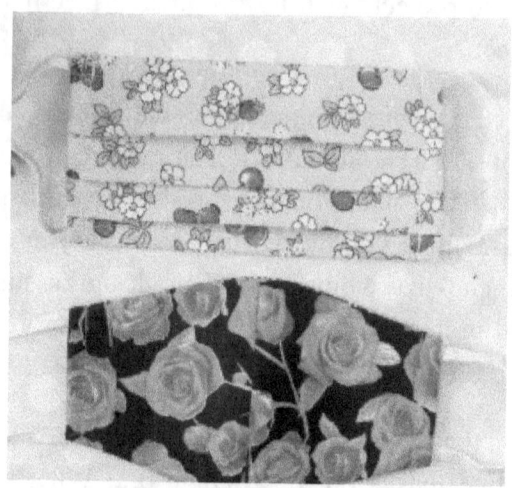

Equipment required:

- Ripper Stitch
- Iron
- Sewing or safety pins
- Ruler
- Needle and thread
- Scissors
- Permanent marker
- 1 medium non-woven polypropylene shopping bag
- 60-inch tape, ½ and 1-inch wide
- 2 pipe cleaners (or plastic-coated belts)

Directions:

1. Check on your shelves for a reusable shopping bag and wash it thoroughly. Avoid disposable plastic and go for reusable non-woven polypropylene shopping bag. This is done putting into consideration the breathability factor. Also, bags coated with foil and plastic material on the inside are not advisable for use. Get the desired bag and especially the one with handles to make things easier. The handles can serve as straps. We shall also get to know how to make straps from the tape in a case where the arms are not long enough for the desired purpose.
2. Cut the edges of the shopping bag to flatten the material and be careful not to cut the handles.
3. Cut the material into two equal sheets. Carefully cut of the seam, if any, at the bottom of the bag. The outcome should be two non-woven polypropylene pages each having its own handle.
4. Measure one of the page and cut a sheet. To establish the middle, use a ruler to measure the edge with a handle. Using a ruler and a marker, locate 4-inch handles with the edge as the starting point. Also, locate 9 inches down from each mark and use your marker to parallel dashed lines and join the line below. Ensure to obtain a 9 by 9 inch square with a top finished edge with handle.
5. Repeat step four for the remaining sheet.
6. Fold over the edge opposite to the handles. Place a sheet with the interior of the initial bag facing upwards and fold half-inch of the material from the edge and iron it. Sew quarter inch from the edge. Load the remaining paper with the outside side of the

initial bag and repeat similar steps to those of the first paper.

Warning: Avoid using extremely high temperature settings when handling the polypropylene type of bags. The use of high ironing temperatures can melt the material. Some iron boxes may lack the poly setting, and therefore, a better option to go for is silk. If the crease isn't set, increase it a little bit. Using an iron box with a desired temperature setting, make each curl.

7. Place the leaves together. The mask will have two layers of fabric. Put one sheet on a clean surface and ensure the stem faces left. Add the second sheet on top of the first one ensuring the handle faces right and secure well. Usually, the printed side should face one direction to ensure a distinction between the front and the back of the mask. It generally ensures proper wearing of the mask.
Fasten the fabric sheets and sew them easily. Get the handles and fold them halfway. Cut the handles in the middle. Test your mask on the face centering it with arms on the sides. The handles should be long and reach out the back of the head with an extra four inches.

8. Make straps out of a ribbon. If handles of the bag in use are short for use, then you have to improvise a better way of creating them. Using a scrapper, remove the handles of the non-woven polypropylene sheet.

Hold the mask at the center of the face and determine the length of each strap using a tape measure. The strap should be long enough to go past the back of the head from the edge of the face. It should simply fit you comfortably. Wear the mask to check on its suitability. If the length of the strip is suitable for use, double the strip and put the pieces on the back of the leaves.

9. Carefully sew the leaves together and double the thread before sewing the edges.
10. Finalize with the edge on the bottom. Make a wrinkle of about ½ inch and iron as in step 6. Remember to sew an inch quarter off the edge.
11. Make a strap that can be adjusted. Fold half an inch of the top edge and iron carefully. Take the pipe cleaners, twist them or the clamps together before cutting a width similar to that of the mask. Fold on the ends to allow fixing. Before fixing them on top, put metal clamps in the fold. Sew the folds of the ligaments and ensure everything is in place. You can go for those ligaments that are accumulated after buying a loaf of bread. This can make a wonderful and functional noseband.
12. Prepare three layers to fold and enlarge the mask. Let the folds be about an inch wide, half an inch on the inner side, and parallel to the nasal fascia. If desired, calibrate the lines on the fabric, fold them and stretch them in position. Then sew a quarter an inch from the edges. Double up the stitch to ensure robustness in the crease. Make three layers in the mask and carefully iron them.

13. Your mask is now ready for use, but before using it, ensure proper sterilization. Soak the mask for a period of 10 minutes in boiling water. If you will need to reuse it, sterilize it well in boiling water.

    It is also important to keep in mind that a mask alone cannot protect fully. Also, protect your eyes with goggles and avoid touching the surface of the mask covering the mouth and nose. Always remember to sterilize your mask after each subsequent use. Ensure it dries well to prevent nurturing an environment suitable for bacterial growth. After every sterilization process, keep your mask in a clean, plastic container.

Mask 3: DIY Child Surgical Mask

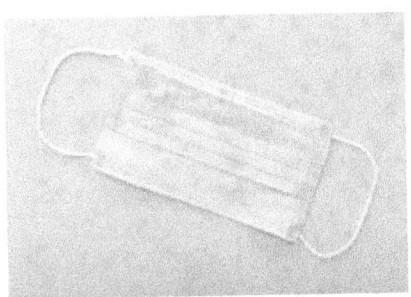

Equipment required:

- Normal Surgical Mask (Adult)
- Double-sided tape

Directions:

1. Identify a unique, fitting, and suitable mask size for your child. If you've already secured one for your child, then it's better to follow the following procedure to understand how you can come up with one. Make a clear comparison of the mask we are going to prepare with the mask already in use.
2. Prepare a crease by folding the extra material of the adult mask.

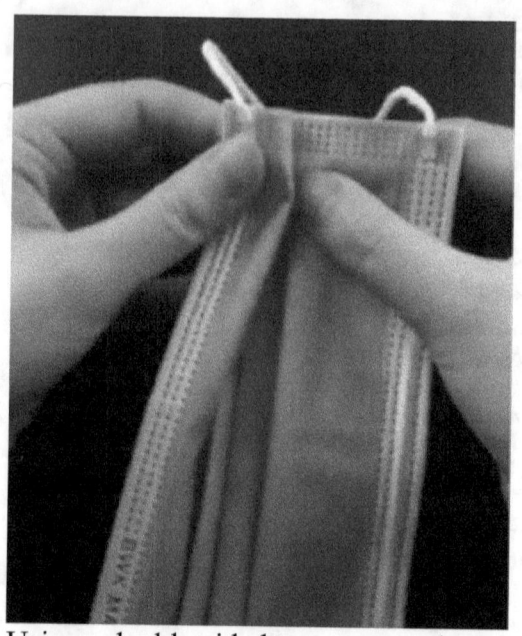

3. Using a double-sided tape, secure the crease.
4. Remove the film from the inside of the mask and fold in the excess material inside your mask.
5. Use another strip of tape to secure well
6. Fold halfway the left side of the material
7. Let the ear loop on the mask face its turn outwards and ensure it fits your child properly. Make a knot in each ear loop and create a snug that fits your child's ear.

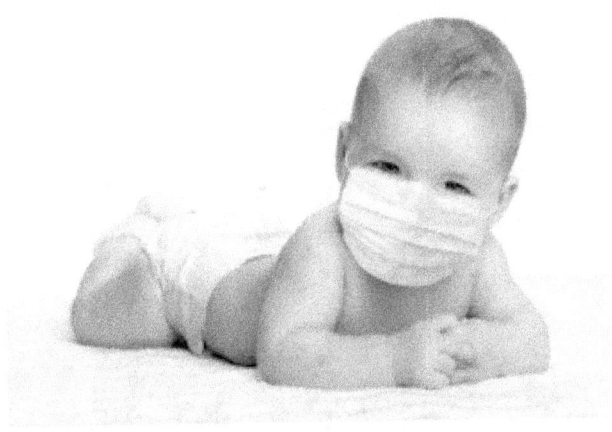

Mask 4: Mask Made of a Napkin

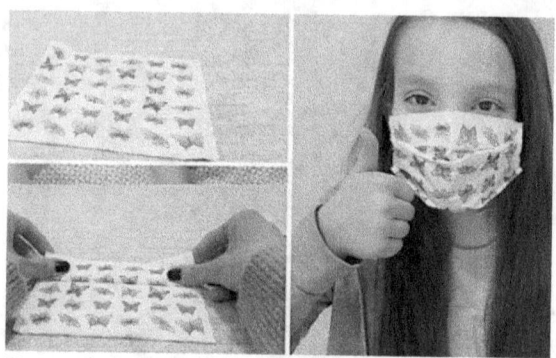

Ever thought of a napkin as a suitable material for your mask? Here is the best way to make a mask from a napkin or paper towel if there isn't anything else.

Equipment's required:
- Clerical Stapler
- Paper Towel
- Two Thin Elastic bands

Directions:

1. First of all, separate a sheet from the already available roll and make folds out of it. Fold with fanfold lines.
2. Put elastic bands on all ends of the sheet.
3. Bend the edge to about 0.4 inches and secure with a stapler to make the elastic band move freely inside. Repeat the same process for the second edge.
4. Enlarge the mask and ensure that it fits you properly. The mask can be replaced from time to time. Cut the tips of the already used mask, release the elastic

bands, and attach a different napkin. Fix everything with a stapler.

Mask 5: Mask made with a gauze

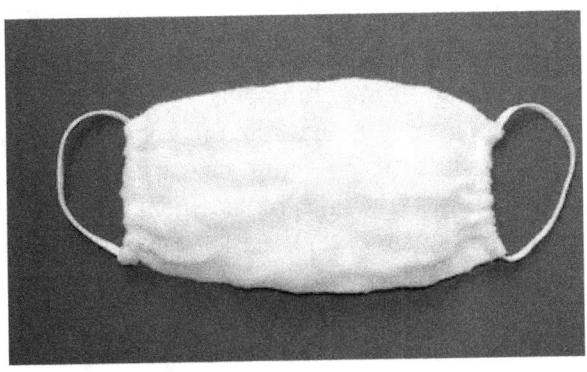

Do you know you can design a proper mask out of a gauze just lying in your house unused? Get your gauze and get set to make a mask for yourself.

Equipment required:
- Ruler
- Needle
- Cotton
- Thread
- Gauze
- Scissors

Directions:

1. Measure a 35.4 by 15.7 inches strip of gauze.
2. Ensure to fold the gauze along the long side.

3. Measure 13.7 inches on both sides and cut them along the middle.
4. A 7.9 inch sided square remains at the center and should form the basis of the anticipated mask. Cut a square of 7.7x7.9 inches from the wool and ensure that it's at least 0.4 inches thick. Put inside the square gauze. Suture on three sides of then basis of the mask to prevent cotton from getting out.

A mask with a wool incorporated in between requires a maximum time of 3-4 hour in use. After that, it should undergo immediate replacement. To enhance its functionality, spray the mask with an antiseptic and wait until it dries.

Mask 6: Double-layer face mask:

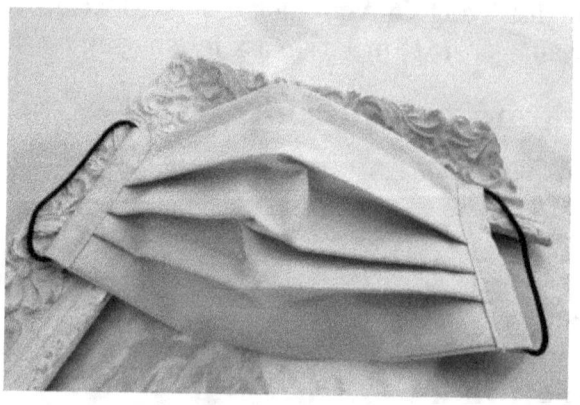

There is a uniqueness that comes with the use of a double-layered face mask. The mask can be worn alternatively. It's not recommendable to alternate the sides in single-use as it can pose a danger of contacting harmful pathogens.

Equipment required:

- Thread
- Paper
- Elastic cord (7 inches)
- Breathable tightly woven fabric (cotton/cotton + polyester)
- Scissors
- Needle or sewing machine

Directions:

1. Get yourself two pieces of cotton fiber and cut them in size 9x7 inches
2. Put one of the pieces on top of the other ensuring that the unsuitable side is outside.
3. Take two 7-inch elastic cords and put one inside the fabric, ensuring both sides near the opposite edges. Repeat the same for the remaining elastic cord.
4. Stitch every edge and leave a 2-inch unstitched part on one of the longest sides. Backstitch at the start and end to prevent from unstitching.
5. From the opening of two inches, turn the mask inside out.
6. Ensure to have a breathing room by making 3 half-inch pleats at regular distances then stitch them.
7. Stitch the opening that had been left initially.
8. You can now use your double-sided, reusable, and washable mask.

9. In the case where your mask is unfitting, adjust the size of the fabric and cords to suit your desire.
10. It is advisable to have three masks of the sought so that one should be for washing after use, one for usage, and another one for backup.

Mask 7: Face mask with filter paper:

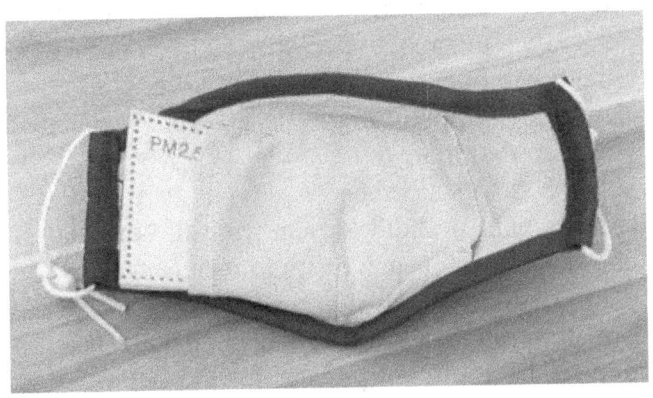

The face mask with filter paper essentially involves a pocket into which a filter is inserted to enhance protection. For more effectiveness, it is advised to change the filters on a regular basis. Also, regular washing practices are advisable.

Equipment required:
- Thread
- Breathable tightly woven fabric
- Two elastic bands 7 inches each
- Scissors
- Needle or sewing machine
- Clips and pins

Directions:

1. Fold the cloth and ensure one of its sides faces the opposite side.
2. Put a paper pattern on the fabric and pin it.

3. Cut the fabric after leaving 3 by 8 inches for the seams. Remember to reserve an inch of fabric on the outer layer and about 0.5 inches on the inner layer.
4. Draw seam lines with tracing paper if possible
5. Turn the fabric over and secure the pair together. Focus on the right.
6. Sew the curves together
7. Draw a line of about ¼ inch from the original seam line and do the same for the other end of the inner seam.
8. Cut the seam allowance about 0.5 inches apart. Repeat the trimming process for the outer and inner layer.
9. Turn the piece over to the right secure the seam allowance, and sew close to the seam line. Do the same for the inner layer and fold the second side of the inner layer next to the original seam line.
10. Sew and repeat the process on both sides of the layer with topstitching.
11. Put the inner layer on top of the outer layer and sew the lower and upper folds in two layers.
12. Cut the seam allowance curve at the meeting point of the two layers approximately 0.5 inches from the edge.
13. Fold the bottom and top of the outer layer twice. Also, fold the seam close to the top. Do the same for the lower seam edge.
14. Leave the rubber at the side pockets and edges. Mark a vertical line and sew with the upper seam border stitch, ensuring to reserve openings at the top and

bottom. Leave openings for inserting rubber bands. The opening can also serve to be a filter opening.
15. Depending on the size and choice, align the elastic band with the pocket mask.
16. A dry antibacterial tissue can serve as a filter in this kind of mask.
17. Always remember to occasionally change the filters, wash the mask frequently, and observe all the hygienic measures when handling the masks.

Mask 8: Surgical/medical face mask

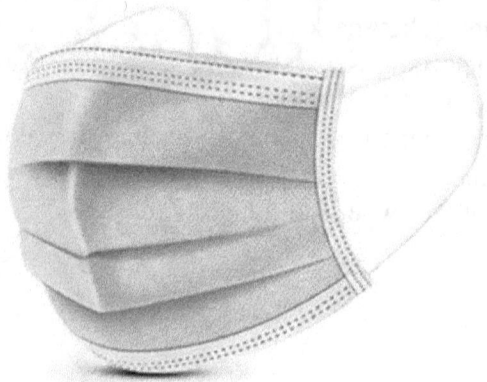

Equipment required:
- Needle or sewing machine
- Paper
- Elastic cord
- Scissors
- Thread
- Breathable tightly woven fabric (cotton/cotton + polyester)

Directions:

1. Get a sizeable piece of paper and cut out a rough surgical mask pattern. Test it on your face and compare its suitability in the mirror. Check to ensure that it fits on your chin, face, and nose. Cut the paper to your liking. Form an exact model of the surgical mask and work towards making even more masks. Reserve the paper for other uses.

2. Put the design on a thick, soft, and breath-friendly fabric. Wash the mask thoroughly to preshrink it. Draw a pattern on the fabric as many times to attain the desired number of face masks. Leave a little more for error accountability.
3. Cut about half-inch of cloth and fold them in halves then sew around the mask edges to ensure even tightness and firmness. Remember to put the breathability factor into consideration.
4. Tightly fix the elastic band onto the surgical mask and wear it around your ears to ensure it is correctly fitting. A number of options are available. You can opt for small elastic cords and thread them on the lower and upper seams of the mask. Always sew the length of the elastic cord to lower and upper masks on the side to enable the creation of a loop.
5. Give a try to your very first surgical mask and make sure you make it rightfully. Always adjust the rubber's length to achieve your desired fit. You can also examine the appearance of your mask and determine its ability to satisfy people using it. There is an instance where the rubber pulls the mask closer to the eyes. In such a case, always cut the cord a little bit to acquire the desired fit.

Mask 9: Gas face mask

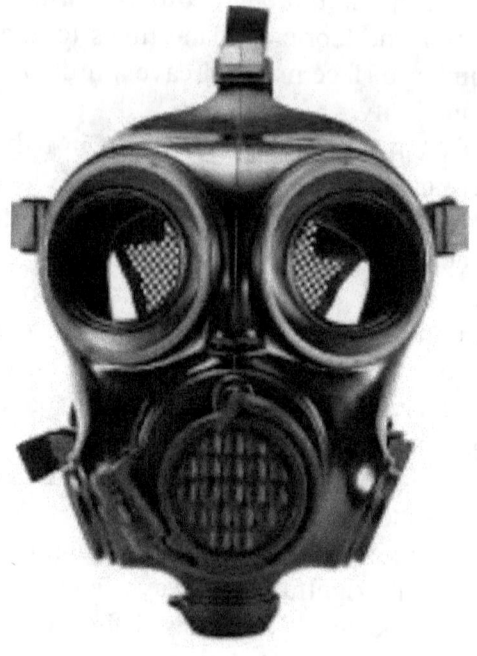

Use of a homemade face masks doesn't guarantee that you will have total protection against pathogens in air and surfaces. But gas face mask definitely has some importance when it comes to situations of haze, smog and smoke. The breathability that comes with use of these masks is quite promising.

Equipment required:
- Duct tape
- A knife
- A 2-liter soda bottle

- A dust mask

Directions:

1. To start off making your gas mask, cut along the seam at the bottom of the 2-liter soda bottle.
2. Scrap off or remove the plastic label on the bottle.
3. Cut a U-shape out of the seam to about 5 cm from the cap of the bottle. You can adjust the width to fit your face perfectly. Always remember that large ones can leave huge gaps that can allow penetration of smoke or spray.
4. Take your dust mask and remove the strap before putting the mask at the bottom of the U-shaped cut out section of the bottle. After placing the mask, a small filter chamber will remain in between the mask and the cap region.
5. Use a strong adhesive tape to fix the mask onto the bottle. Add some tape along the bottle's jagged edges. Use duct tape enhances comfort provided by the mask and also brings some form of smoothness to when using it.
6. Make several slits around the top of the mask and one slit on each of the sides. Cut about 2 inches below and make two additional slits on each side.
7. Pass and thread a rubber band through the slots and tie them with a flat knot.
8. Put some more tape on the slots to prevent air from penetrating into the mask.
9. Make more holes to enhance and facilitate breathability

Mask 10: Handkerchief or Bandana Face mask

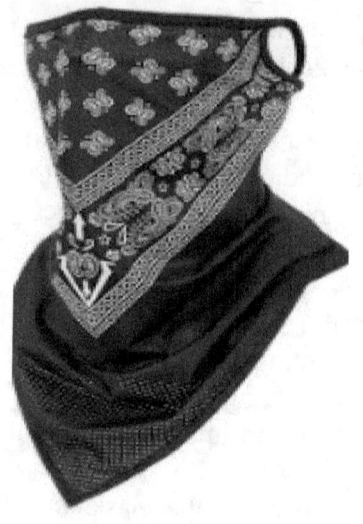

Equipment required:

- Scissors
- Bandana or handkerchief
- Hair ties
- Coffee filter

Directions:

1. Start off by cutting the coffee filter halfway and longitudinally.

2. Put the already cut filter paper in the midst through a bandana or handkerchief.

3. Turn top and bottom of the bandana over the centered paper.

4. Put hair ties on either side of the coffee filter ensuring a separation distance of about 7 inches.

5. Tuck in the sides of the bandana into the hair ties

6. Ensure to sterilize your mask before using it

Mask 11: Face mask with cricut

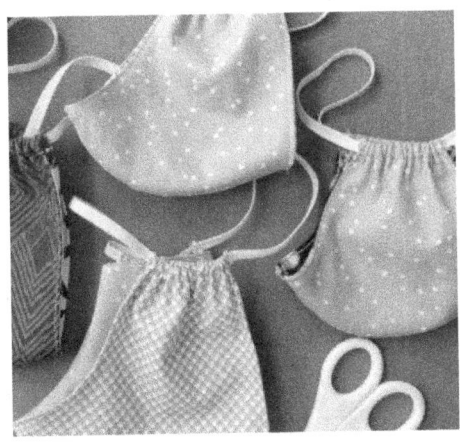

Equipments required:

- Small safety pin
- Scissors
- Cushion for Fabric Grip fabric
- 6 mm (¼") braided elastic
- Pen in washable fabric
- Bray
- Cricut Maker
- Rotary mulch

The fabric you choose:

- For the internal fabric, measure 7 x 16 inches.
- For the external fabric, measure 8 by 16 inches

Directions:

1. To adjust some things in this project, move parts of different mats or colors using opaque preview screen. Usually, it's advisable to turn the parts without altering the arrangement so that the feel and texture of the fabric is retained.

2. Preshrink the fabric by thoroughly washing it. Alternatively, you can press it with non-washable steam and cut it.

3. Cut the fabric and reserve it on the mat. Identify the direction of the grain for each fabric piece.

4. Put together all the pieces and press them if there is need.

5. Join the dark blue outer pieces together with right sides and sew the curved part with ¼ inch stitch. Do the same for the inside and cut along the curve while ensuring not to cut the seam.

6. Press the flat edges about 6 millimeters down the liner edge.

7. Carefully sew the edge of the lining piece

8. Press the border plates about ¼ inch down right from the edge of the coating.

9. Fold the outside and press it to form elastic band housing. Sew close to the pre-printed edge to leave enough space.

10. Press the curved seam on one of the sides and the top seam along the side of the curved seam of each outer and lining part.

11. Press the curved seam on one side and the top seam along this side of the curved seam of each outer and lining part.

12. Align the parts and sides to the right and sew with a 6-millimeter stitch along the top and bottom. Stretch the stitches to ensure they are firm and stiff.

13. Cut off the edges if necessary. Turn one of the side openings and press all the points. Reinforce the upper seams along the top and bottom.

14. Use a small safety pin to thread the rubber band over the bottom box on one side. Thread towards the other side of the mask until it meets the other end of the elastic band.

15. Secure the elastic with a zigzag stitch and ensure no twisting occurs in the elastic. Put the elastic seam on the body to ensure proper comfort.

16. If necessary, insert a filter into the mask via the openings on the side, and your mask will be ready for use.

Mask 12: Easy No-Sew Face Mask

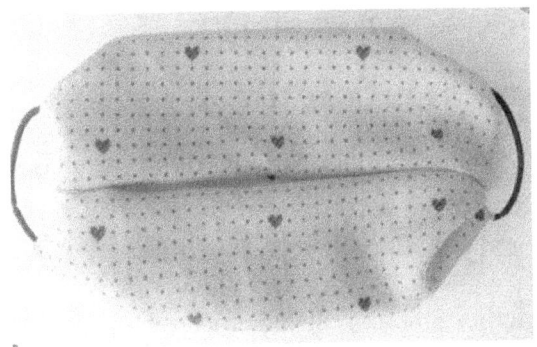

Do you have no skills in sewing? Don't get worried. The easy no sew face mask is the best through way for you. The design of this mask is the simplest and easiest as it requires no time for sewing, and no sewing skills are required. Just a couple of minutes, and your mask can be considered ready for use. The goodness with this kind of mask is that it incorporates the use of a few reusable and washable materials. However, the mask doesn't use effective materials fit for shielding the wearer against pathogens. It is, therefore, essential to include filter material into your mask. Materials used are easily accessible; hence no need for straining to look for materials that aren't easily available. The filter is the only material you will have to look for. Considering critical times of pandemic, it is easier to source the filter than accessing a surgical mask. The easy no-sew face masks cone with advantages, and among them is the ability to adjust it to the desired size.

Equipment required:

- A sizeable handkerchief of any material. Any size can do better but consider having smaller ones for children and the larger ones for grownups.

- Two stretchy spare hair elastics for each mask.

- Scissors,

- Some Electrostatic filter paper

Directions:

1. Prepare the surface you will be working on by thoroughly cleaning it and disinfecting it. Do the same for the equipment you'll be using. Ensure to wash your hands after the cleaning process and avoid touching the material until when your hands are clean.

2. Put your filter paper out and measure out a piece of it to fit your nose and mouth. Cut a single piece for each face mask you are about to make and reserve it with the remaining filter paper.

3. Put your handkerchief flat and open on your working surface. Align it so that it resembles a square or diamond facing your direction. You can alternatively put the filter paper in a different location and fold it accordingly. If you are using the square shape, put the already cut filter paper in the middle of the handkerchief. First, fold the top over the filter paper then fold the bottom over to attain a long, even rectangular shape. If you use the diamond shape, put the filter close to the top corner. Fold the top corner down to the center of the diamond and also fold over the filter paper. Fold the bottom corner towards the middle to ensure the two corners touch each other. Fold the handkerchief from top to bottom to acquire a regular shape.

4. Regardless of the shape used, you can add hair elastics. Put the hair elastic over each end of the already folded handkerchief and pull it towards the middle. The hair elastics can be used to adjust the size of the mask. Pull the hair elastics closer to the middle to ensure proper fitting for children. Otherwise, pull them away from the middle to ensure that they

properly fit the adults. These hair elastics serve as ear loops and keeps the mask intact on the face whenever in use. Ensure they are stretchy to enhance comfortability.

5. After adjusting the hair elastics to your desired level of comfortability, fold the handkerchief ends towards the middle. If the handkerchief is too long, you can fold each end into each other to ensure they hold in place. In a case where they are short, you can fold each side in on itself and tuck all the ends under the hair elastic. By doing so, you will be able to remove the filter paper and replace it with a new one. To enhance the effectiveness of your mask, use some adhesive tape to hold the ends in place. Ensure all the ends are firm. Your mask is now ready for use, and you can easily adjust the straps whenever you want to do so.

The design used in making this kind of mask is basically simple and easy. Therefore, anyone with the required materials can make it whenever the need arises. The use of filter material in this kind of mask enhances its suitability by providing an extra protection mechanism against dangerous pathogens. The mask can, therefore, achieve a higher protection level against smaller and larger harmful droplets.

Alternative materials can be used as a replacement for the handkerchief. A relatively large scarf can also be a better substitute for the handkerchief. With a scarf, about 43% protection capability can be achieved. The use of filters can enhance effectiveness by about double the rate. Masks without filters tend to lower the level of protection by allowing more harmful particles to penetrate through the mask. But also a scarf without a filter paper can work well compared to a handkerchief without a filter paper. The advantage of using a handkerchief is that it makes your work easier. Scarfs can be made from a variety of materials, of which some materials can only be good for use.

Always use a filter paper, and if it is inaccessible, you can opt to use a double layer of handkerchiefs for this kind of design. Always work towards enhancing protection provided by the mask.

Mask 13: Using Paper Towels to Make Face Mask

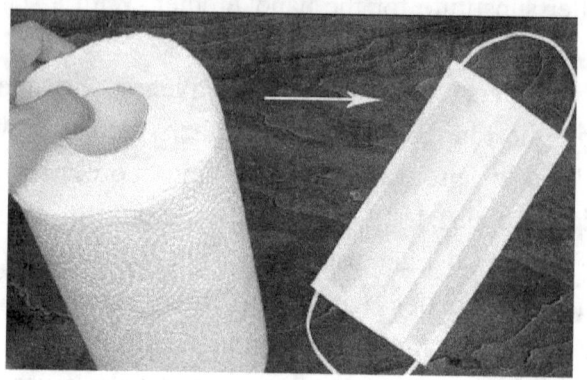

Equipment required:

- Rubber Band,
- Paper Towel,
- Stapler,
- Scissors

Directions:

1. Get a piece of paper towel and cut a sizeable piece. Ensure the size is twice the mask you want to make. The masks we want to prepare are of dimensions 6 by 5 inches. Therefore, you will have to cut paper towels of size 6 by 6 inches.

2. Fold the paper towel into half to acquire a rectangular shape of dimensions 6 by 5 inches.

3. Make pleats or folds that are parallel to the rectangle's longest end. Ensure each fold is around an inch away from the initial fold.

4. Always ensure that every fold goes in the same direction as the initial fold. Ensure to obtain a zigzag pattern.

5. Continue to fold towards the of the paper towel. Ensure you reach the utmost end.

6. Carefully hold the folds in position

7. Make a small fold across the left side and put a single rubber band underneath. Use a stapler to fasten it. Staple twice to ensure the band is firmly secured.

8. Follow the same steps for the right side of the paper towel.

9. Unfold the ready mask and use it with strict usage precautions.

Mask 14: Homemade Cotton fabric face mask

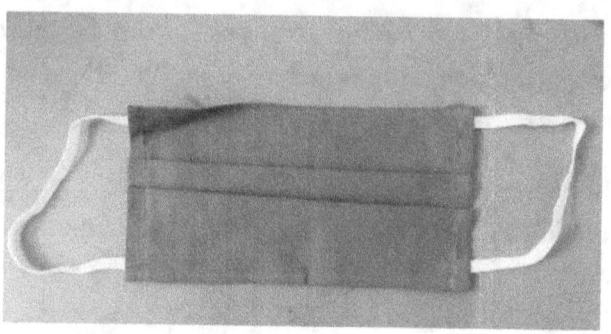

Equipment required:

- A piece of cotton fabric,
- Measuring tape,
- Sewing machine or thread and needle,
- Scissors, elastic band, and
- Sewing pins

Directions:

1. Cut the cotton fabric into two square pieces, each with size 7 by 7 inches.

2. Put each fabric piece such that its front or public side faces the pubic side of the opposite piece. By doing

so, the fabrics will appear in such a way that their insides are out.

3. Sew the edges on the side and also do the same for the fabrics. Sew them together.

4. Unwrap the fabrics by taking the insides back. Ensure the wefts' sides are outside.

5. Make folds or pleats ensuring that they are about half an inch apart at the center of the fabrics. Use the sewing pins to secure the folds or pleats in place. You now sew.

6. All pleats or folds can either be made in the same directions or should go in different directions. But if you choose to use different directions, ensure that all pleats add up to an even number.

7. The bottom half of the pleats should face the top edge of the fabric. The top half of the pleats should be made to point towards the bottom edge of the fabric.

8. Sew the right and left sides of the fabric and hold the pleats in position.

9. Make a helm on both sides of the fabric then leave the top and bottom of the hem open.

10. Prepare two pieces from the elastic band, ensuring that each piece is approximately 7 inches long.

11. Put one end of the elastic band into the bottom opening on the left side hem of the fabric. Sew the using the running stitch and ensure its firmly into position.

12. Use the remaining end of the same piece of elastic band. Sew it into the top opening of the left side hem.

13. Use the other piece of elastic band and fix it on the right side hem. To do so, you can refer to the procedure above.

14. The mask is now ready for use. It is washable, reusable, and efficient. Only stick to the usage strategies to achieve the best results.

Mask 15: Home Made Mask with a Filter Pocket

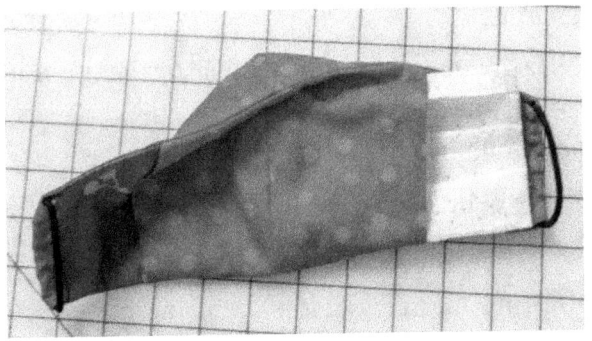

Equipment required:

- 1 Piece of flannel for the middle layer (6" x9")
- 2 pieces of material - cotton is best (6" x 9")
- 2 pieces of elastic. The thinner, the better as it is way more comfortable.
- Pins to hold down the fabric
- Pair of scissors

Directions:

1. Get the flannel piece of cloth and put it flat on your work area.

2. Use the cotton fabric on the outside or rather use a preferable piece for your mask. Put it over the flannel fabric.

3. Use a single piece of the elastics and pin it on the top of the fabric that's flat on the surface. The elastic should be about half inch when tucked. Ensure it is on the top right corner. Pin it firmly to ensure it is secured in place.

4. Bring the remaining side of the elastic to the bottom of the fabric on the surface. The stretchy material will serve as one of the straps that will extend to the left ear. Ensure to firmly pin it down. You will also have to ensure that the elastic is half-inch when tucked. Mark equal distances from the top to the bottom.

5. Fix the elastic to the other side and create a strap for the mask. Ensure that it goes over to the left ear.

6. You can use the other piece of cotton to serve as a lining fabric. You can go on to put it over everything that's already on your work area. Ensure to have your flannel as the first layer, and the cotton should serve as the second layer. The elastic should be attached with pins, then add the second piece of cloth on top.

7. You can now clip everything once again to ensure that the fabrics are attached. Ensure you hold down the elastic in position to ensure firmness.

8. After re-clipping everything, you will now need to take everything to a sewing machine. Alternatively, you can use a needle a thread to sew carefully. You can also opt to use a ¼ seam to enhance the results. Stitch all the sides together and double stitch the elastic bands to ensure it is firmly secured.

9. The use of a sewing machine should be accompanied by some precautions. Ensure to leave the seam open so that you can add extra filters.

10. After finishing the sewing process, you will now be approaching the completion of your mask. You can opt to slightly trim the edges of your mask, being careful not to destroy the elastic. By doing so, you will be enhancing the comfortability provided by the mask.

11. With the seam open, you can opt to turn the mask from inside anytime you want. You can also turn it over according to your desire. You can now start getting assured of the effectiveness of a homemade mask.

12. To achieve even better results, you can push out the corners using your fingers or a pen with a cap on.

13. Remember to note the side with the opening. Use your iron to carefully press the fabric. Through ironing, the material becomes straight and neater.

14. After ironing, hold the top of the mask and fold it down. By folding down, you will achieve the resemblance of folds found in some given masks. A three-inch fold can be better off. You can, therefore, clip the ends and prepare for stitching.

15. Repeat the same by folding lower down your mask to have about two folds. Pin it down to prepare it for stitching. Ensure its about 3 inches.

16. You can now take your iron and press it for a short time and ensure to regulate the heat accordingly. High heat levels can burn your mask and destroy the whole process.

17. Lastly, you can now stitch all the areas to give more accommodation for the folds. Ensure all the folds are permanently done. Stitching will also be essential for the initially created seam.

18. You can now decide on whether to leave the seam open or add extra protection to enhance the efficiency

of the mask. If your choice is to have additional protection, you can go for the most efficient filters.

At this point, you can now consider having created a completely secure mask. Ensure to open your mask up to enhance its efficiency and comfortability on the mouth and nose. Also, ensure to use the desired measurements so that the mask fits almost every size of the face.

The use of various colors can also produce varied results that can help you identify the best mask. The masks are very easy to make provided that accessibility to desired materials is guaranteed. Even when you don't have a sewing machine, you really don't have to stress yourself because a regular thread and needle can do. So, it's not a must to use a sewing machine in cases where sewing is required.

The benefits that come with the use of the above masks are summarized below.

- There is greater protection offered since the mask has a total of three layers.

- Leaving the seam open gives you an option of using filters to enhance the protection provided by the mask.

- Materials are cheap and can be easily accessed
- Masks can be prepared from a range of materials with different colors
- In the unavailability of N95 masks, protective gear can be used by medical personnel as an alternative.

These are some of the easiest, quickest and achievable methods you can use to design a range of protective masks. The masks are more efficient and economical as there is the consideration of aspects of washing and reusability. Some of them have filters incorporated in them to enhance their effectiveness while in use. The use of filters requires frequent changes after every usage. Generally, handle them cautiously and adhere to washing hands before and after using the masks. It is also good to avoid close contacts with surfaces of already used masks.

Conclusion

The use of homemade face masks is essential as it comes with several key advantages. Cost-effectiveness and eco-friendliness are just but some of the advantages you will achieve with the use of homemade face masks. The medical experts and professionals find a hard time to handle a range of patients with harmful diseases such as coronavirus. It is, therefore, important to shield them by ensuring that they have enough protective masks of the type N95. But to achieve this, the design of a homemade mask is essential. With an influx of these masks on the market, there is an increased chance of protection to both the health personnel and the world at large. Currently, the world is faced with threats from multiple epidemics that rise day and night. We have seen many falling victims of the viruses, and many have lost lives just because of these new diseases. We are therefore required to explore many strategies to minimize the spread of these diseases worldwide. One of the ways is making effective homemade masks. Let us focus on protecting ourselves and others. If we manage to protect ourselves, we can extend the protection to the person next to us, and finally nations and nations worldwide. Always adhere to strategies and rules that govern the effective use of masks and enhance the protection rate. With disease threats arising, many people will flood stores to buy masks as a way of preventing the spread of diseases such as the coronavirus. As a result, there can be the inadequacy of masks in the market, and you will not need to struggle. The best option is to design your face masks of your own.

The use of masks designed at home doesn't guarantee that you will receive total protection against pathogens on surfaces and in air. But consider having no mask at all. With no mask, you will have a higher risk of contracting these diseases and spreading them to other people. You will also need to understand fabrics and filters to ensure you come up with the best mask ever. Apart from protecting the spread of dangerous airborne diseases, masks can also be essential in other areas. Apart from protection from the contraction of viral and bacterial infections, masks are also essential in protecting personalities during seasonal changes. The society should, therefore, be geared towards protecting the whole world before diseases become fatal.

You will need to have these facemasks for the security of your family. So if you can't access one, don't panic, don't be anxious and don't be afraid. Don't even move from one store to another yearning to get at least a mask for your family. Sit down at the comfort of home, design your D.I.Y mask from your materials, and protect yourself and the people around you. Source out the desired materials and settle your problems concerning masks.

The mask designs explored in this book are customizable, suitable, and fit for any age. Items used in many of the masks are easily accessible; hence no need for straining to seek special materials. Therefore, keep calm and settle down because your problems are already solved.

www.ingramcontent.com/pod-product-compliance
Lightning Source LLC
Chambersburg PA
CBHW070253220526
45465CB00004B/1608